ECG & EKG Interpretation

How to interpret ECG & EKG, including rhythms, arrhythmias, and more!

Copyright 2015

Table of Contents

Introduction 1

Chapter 1: Introduction to Electrocardiogram 2

Chapter 2: Understanding the Conduction System of the Heart.. 7

Chapter 3: Learning the Basics of ECG Interpretation............ 11

Chapter 4: Interpreting Normal ECG Readings 15

Chapter 5: Recognizing Arrhythmias...................................... 21

Chapter 6: Caring for the Heart 25

Conclusion 28

Introduction

I want to thank you and congratulate you for downloading the book, "ECG & EKG Interpretation".

This book contains helpful information about an ECG, what it is, and how to read one!

Learning about ECG scans will help you to better understand the ECG results of yourself and others. Through reading this book, you will learn about how the heart functions, and the various things that can go wrong in the heart.

This book includes great tips and techniques that will help you to better understand the ECG/EKG, and interpret it correctly. This includes teaching you how to identify when an ECG scan looks irregular.

You will learn about the different irregularities that can occur, and what each of them looks like on an ECG scan paper.

Lastly, you will be given some great strategies to help improve the health of your heart. Being able to understand the results of an ECG is a good skill, but it's even more important to ensure that the results you receive are good ones!

Thanks again for downloading this book, I hope you enjoy it!

Chapter 1:
Introduction to Electrocardiogram

The heart is a unique organ. Each beat is accomplished by the synchronized activities of these three: the electrical impulses flowing through a nodal tissue pathway in the heart, the muscles of the heart and the valves of the heart. Any deviation from the normal of these three factors will affect the pace or rhythm of the heart, which in turn, will affect the overall cardiovascular system. On the other hand, any alteration or abnormality in the cardiovascular system will create a great negative impact on the general health of the person; hence, it is vital to assess this electrical activity regularly. That is where ECG or EKG comes in.

What is ECG or EKG?

Electrocardiogram (ECG) or (EKG) is a painless, non-invasive procedure primarily used to determine the electrical activity of the heart. At the same time, it can also determine the following:

- Rate and rhythm of the heart

- Presence of ischemia (inadequate blood supply)

- Causative factors of angina or chest pain, palpitations, shortness of breath, dizziness and fainting spells

- Occurrence of a heart attack

- Condition of the chambers of the heart (whether there is hypertrophy or enlargement)

- Structural irregularities of the valves of the heart such as presence of obstructions, holes or narrowing (stenosis)

Aside from these, ECG is also useful because it performs the following functions:

- Ascertain if the prescribed cardiac medicines are working

- Determine if an implanted device, such as a pacemaker, is functioning accordingly

- Monitor the health of the heart of those individuals who are prone to developing cardiac diseases due to genetics and unhealthy lifestyle

How is the procedure done?

A doctor, nurse or ECG technician can perform ECG to a person, whether as an inpatient or outpatient. No special preparation is required for this exam. However, to ensure the accuracy of the results, it is advisable to do the following before undergoing the procedure:

1. There should be no intake of any medicines (for example, cardiac and antidepressant drugs) that may alter the results of ECG.

2. There should be no intake of any stimulants, such as sodas, coffee or teas, as these are known to affect the rate and rhythm of the heart.

3. There should be no rigorous or heavy workout or activity prior to the exam. The patient should be well rested.

Materials to prepare:

- ECG machine
- ECG strip or paper
- Sticky pads for the electrodes
- Wipes
- Razor (in case the patient has hairy chest)

Step-by-step guide to do a standard (also known as routine or resting) ECG procedure

1. Check the doctor's order. Explain the procedure to the patient.
2. Provide privacy. Properly screen the bed or close the door. A companion is allowed according to the patient's preference.
3. Wash hands.
4. Assist the patient in removing his or her top shirt.
5. Place the patient in supine or lying position. If the patient is having difficulty in breathing or is unable to

assume this position, a semi-Fowler's position (slightly upright position) is also acceptable.

6. If the patient's chest is hairy, shaving it off is sometimes required to ensure accurate results.

7. Place the 10 electrodes according to the standardized system – six electrodes on the chest wall and four electrodes on the extremities. Here is the proper placement on the chest wall and the color code:

	Location	Color Code
V1	4th intercostal space, right sternal edge	brown/red
V2	4th intercostal space, left sternal edge	brown/yellow
V3	mid-way between v2 and V4	brown/green
V4	5th intercostal space, mid-clavicular line	brown/blue
V5	5th intercostal space, anterior axillary line	brown/orange
V6	5th intercostal space, horizontal mid axillary line	brown/purple

For the extremities, the color code is red (for the left leg), green (right leg), black (left arm) and white (right arm).

It is very important that the electrodes are properly attached, as misplaced electrodes will produce inaccurate results. At the same time, it is important to instruct the patient to remain still while undergoing the procedure. A slight movement can interfere with the tracing of the electrical activity of the heart.

8. Press the start button of the ECG machine. It will start to record and translate on the ECG paper or strip the electrical activity of the heart.

9. Write the name of the patient, date and time of the procedure on the ECG paper.

10. Remove the electrodes. Clean the sticky areas with wipes.

At this point, one can scan the results of the ECG. If one is knowledgeable in interpreting ECG, then he or she will be able to know the rate, rhythm and condition of the heart (to a certain degree) even prior to the release of the official written result. This is easily learned when one has full comprehension of the conduction system of the heart. What is this? Find out in the proceeding chapter.

Chapter 2:
Understanding the Conduction System of the Heart

The heart pumps oxygenated blood throughout the body. To be able to do that, it needs a power source such as electricity. This is similar to a regular pump machine that works on electricity, too. The difference is that the heart creates its own electrical impulses, then it controls these impulses through a special conduction pathway. This is known as the conduction system of the heart.

Even when the heart is outside the body and even without the input of the nervous system, it will continue to beat as long as the specialized myocardial cells are alive and the conduction system is working.

How does the conduction system take place?

The conduction system is made possible by the automaticity property of the heart. This simply means that the creation and use of the electrical impulses is spontaneous. There is no need for any stimulus or interference from other body systems to initiate the electrical activity of the heart.

As mentioned, to produce a single beat, the muscle activity of the heart (giving the pressure differential needed for the valves) and the movement of the valves (closing and opening) together with the conduction system should be in one accord.

To be able to appreciate the conduction pathway, a brief review of the heart's anatomy and physiology is a must.

The Cardiovascular System

The heart, a muscular organ, is made up of 4 chambers. The chambers consist of two atria (left and right) on the upper half of the heart and two ventricles (left and right) on the lower half. Separating the atria from the ventricles are the valves. On the other hand, the septum divides the atria and ventricles from left and right.

The heart works together with the respiratory and vascular systems to convert deoxygenated blood to oxygenated blood. This then will be distributed, first to the vital organs and then to the rest of the body.

The blood flow of the heart

Blood travels in a unidirectional way, which simply means in one direction only. The valves prevent the blood from going back to where it has been. Beginning from the upper chamber of the heart, called the right atrium, deoxygenated blood from the head, neck and upper extremities enters the heart through the superior vena cava. In the same manner, blood from the lower extremities and lower parts of the body enters this chamber via the inferior vena cava. Lastly, deoxygenated blood from the heart enters the heart through the coronary sinus.

From there, it will enter the right ventricle by passing through the tricuspid valve. Once the blood enters the right ventricle, backflow to the right atrium is prevented with the help of the tricuspid valve. From the right ventricle, it will enter the lungs through the pulmonary artery. Take note that this is the only artery that carries oxygen deprived blood. In the lungs, gas exchange takes place. The carbon dioxide is released while oxygen is absorbed; thus, the deoxygenated blood turns into oxygenated blood.

The oxygenated blood returns to the heart (specifically to the left atrium) via the pulmonary vein. This is the only vein that carries oxygen rich blood. From the left atrium, it passes through the bicuspid valve going to the left ventricle. Similar to the tricuspid valve, this valve also prevents the backflow of the blood. In the left ventricle, oxygenated blood passes through the semilunar aortic valve going to the aorta. From there, it is distributed into systemic circulation.

The heart pumps an estimated 5-6 liters of blood per minute. This is equivalent to 7200 to 8640 liters of blood in a day. In order to do this, the heart needs to beat at 80-100 beats per minute in a normal adult and around 120-160 beats to infants and young children. How then is the beat produced? An electric impulse is necessary and this is through the conduction system.

The pathway of the conduction system

The good thing is the heart has the ability to make its own electrical impulses. First, the SA (sino-atrial) node, located near the superior vena cava and known as the heart's pacemaker, initiates an impulse. The impulse travels from the upper chamber to the AV (atrioventricular) node, which is located on top of the tricuspid valve. From there, the impulse travels to the bundle of His, which has left and right bundles. The last destination of this electrical impulse is the Purkinje fibers. This results in one rhythmic heartbeat.

There are medical conditions that can prevent the initiation of the impulse at the SA node. When this occurs, the heart tries to compensate by allowing the AV node to initiate the impulse. However, unlike the SA node, which has the capacity to generate impulses at 80-100 times per minute, the AV node can only do as much as 40 to 60 impulses per minute. Still, the body will be able to survive at this rate.

When the AV node fails to deliver the impulses, the bundle of His takes charge. Unfortunately, its ability is up to 20-40 impulses per minute only. Finally, if everything else fails, the Purkinje fiber takes over, with 0-20 impulses only. At this point, the body could give in and not survive.

ECG and the conduction system

Through the ECG procedure, one will be able to determine the condition of the conduction system of the heart. It can reveal where the impulse is being initiated. Is it at the SA node or somewhere else? It can show which part of the conduction pathway has problems or irregularities. It can also detect errors in the rate and rhythm of the heart.

Learn the basics of ECG interpretation in the proceeding chapters.

Chapter 3:
Learning the Basics of ECG Interpretation

Practice is essential in mastering ECG interpretation. It takes patience too to know and understand all the details about ECG interpretation. One needs to memorize numbers, nomenclatures, shapes (deflections) and significance of each shape or tracing. However, when one knows the principles, interpreting becomes easy.

The first important step in achieving the skill on interpreting ECG tests is studying the features of the ECG paper.

ECG paper or strip

ECG paper is a special graph paper. This paper is divided into 1 mm² grid-like boxes. The vertical axis measures the plot voltage while the horizontal axis measures the time. Each small horizontal box (1 mm) corresponds to 0.04 second. Five small boxes will form a large box written in a heavier line. Multiplying the small boxes (with 0.04 second each) into 5, one will come up with 0.20. Therefore, one big box corresponds to 0.20 seconds. Using this formula, 5 big boxes will result to 1 second.

At the top of the ECG paper, there are black marks at 3-second intervals. One can use this as a guide later on when interpreting the results.

Each large box has 5 small boxes high and 5 small boxes long, giving a total of 25 small boxes per big box.

The vertical axis is about amplitude or voltage. Two large boxes correspond to 1 millivolt (mV); therefore, one small box is 0.1 mV. The height of the ECG paper is equivalent to 10 boxes.

ECG Nomenclature

The electrical activity of the heart is also translated into waveform components on the ECG paper after the test. These are labeled with the following letters – P, Q, R, S, T and U.

Each wave represents a specific action of the heart. By counting the boxes, one can determine if the deflection of each wave is within the normal range or not. Also, observe the shapes of the deflections, as they can tell the status of the conduction system to a certain degree.

Using Lead II, here are the waves, complex, segment and intervals that one should expect to see in a normal ECG reading.

1. P wave. It is the first positive deflection, which is usually smooth and round in appearance. It represents atrial depolarization or contraction. The amplitude or voltage along the vertical axis is normally at 0.05 to 0.25mV. This means that if the height of the deflection is from half to 2 1/12 small boxes, it is still within the normal range. The horizontal axis, on the other hand, is in normal range too when it covers 1.5 to 2.75 small boxes. In time, that is 0.06 to 0.11 seconds.

   When looking at the P waves, try to answer the following questions.

   a. Are the P waves present? Check if there is a P wave before every QRS complex. Absence of P waves is an indication that there is an improper, or worse, no contraction, of the atrium.

b. Is there a regular occurrence of P waves? Intermittent (on and off) appearance of P waves is not a good sign of atrial contraction.

c. How do the waves look? Are they in an upright position (positive deflection), rounded and smooth? Are they uniform in appearance?

2. QRS complex. The complex starts with the Q wave on a negative deflection, followed by the R wave on a positive deflection and ends with the S wave on a downward or negative deflection. It represents the contractions of the ventricles. Horizontally, it covers 1.5 to 3 boxes. That is equivalent to 0.06 to 0.12 seconds. Again, observe if the QRS complexes are present and if they look the same.

3. PR Interval. This measures the period from the start of atrial contraction (P wave) until the start of ventricular contraction (R wave from the QRS complex). In other words, it is the AV conduction time. It is equivalent to 3-5 small boxes or 01.2 to 0.20 seconds. With an increased heart rate, this interval is expected to be shorter.

4. T wave. Positioned in a positive deflection, this wave represents ventricular repolarization (resting of the ventricles). After the QRS complex, there is a small pause then followed by the T wave. Absence of T waves is indicative of no rest for the ventricles.

5. QT Interval. This interval is all about ventricular activity – from its contraction until its rest. The measurement starts from the beginning of the QRS complex until the end of the T wave.

6. ST segment. The S wave represents the end of the ventricular contraction while the T wave is the ventricular rest; therefore, this measures the early part of the resting phase of the ventricles. It is usually flat in appearance.

7. U wave. This is the smaller positively deflected wave just after the T wave. In some cases, the U wave does not appear. That is normal and not something to worry about. U wave represents recovery of the Purkinje fibers.

Chapter 4:
Interpreting Normal ECG Readings

As a beginner in interpreting ECG, Lead II is commonly used to interpret the result of ECG; hence, all discussions here are in referral to Lead II. After the ECG procedure, one can determine the following using the ECG result:

- Rate

- Rhythm

- Atrial contraction

- Ventricular contraction

- Atriventricular conduction time

- Ventricular rest or repolarization

- Arrhythmias

- Presence of medical condition or emergency

Checking the Rhythm

A rhythm is a particular pattern. When it comes to the heart, any gross disruption in the rhythm can cause a ripple effect to the systemic circulation.

One can check the rhythm by examining the R-to-R interval. There should be an equal space on all the R-to-R intervals. A margin of 10% variation is still considered within normal. Assess if the rhythm is regular. Atrial rhythm can be checked by measuring the P-to-P interval instead. When checking the rhythm on the ECG paper, there are two methods that one can use. Here they are:

1. The paper and pencil method. Get a piece of paper. Place it against the ECG paper and put a mark on the paper where the first R is. Without moving the paper and ECG paper, mark the second R. Using the marked paper, check all the R-R intervals on the ECG strip. A normal result would show an equal distance on all the R-to-R intervals. It means the rhythm is regular.

2. The caliper method. Set the caliper on the first R on the ECG strip. Next, set the other part of the caliper to the second R. Secure the caliper so that the result will be accurate. Afterwards, measure the rest of the R-R intervals. Check for regularity or consistency. When the set caliper is not the same for the other intervals, it is an indication that the rhythm is not regular.

Checking the Rate

Rate measures the beats of the heart per minute. There are different normal values of heart rate according to age.

For adults, the normal heart rate is at 60-100 beats per minute. A heart rate more than 100 beats/min is termed as tachycardia. A heart rate lower than 100 beats/min is called bradycardia.

For children, here is the guide:

- 0-12 months– 100-160 beats/minute
- 1- 2 years old – 90-150 beats/minute
- 3-5 years old – 80-140 beats/minute
- 6-12 years old – 70-120 beats/minute
- 13 and above - same as the adults

There are several ways to determine heart rate through the ECG strip.

1. The first method involves locating the 6-second interval in the ECG strip. If you recall, one big box is equivalent to 1 second; therefore, 6 seconds would mean six big boxes. Count all the QRS complexes in this 6-second interval. Multiply the results by 10. The product is the heart rate. For example, if there were 7 QRS complexes in the 6-second interval, then 7 x 10 = 70. The heart rate is 70. Regardless whether the rhythm is regular or not, one can use this method to check the heart rate.

2. Using the second method, get one R-to-R interval. Count the number of small boxes from one R wave to the next R wave. Divide the number of small boxes counted into 1500. Round off to the nearest 10. The result is the heart rate. Say there are 22 small boxes in one R-to-R interval so 1500/22. The answer is 68.18. The heart rate is therefore 68 beats per min.

3. Another method uses the R-to-R interval also. This time, count the big boxes within the 2 consecutive R waves. Divide the results to 300. For example, there are 5 large boxes between the first R and the next R wave. The heart rate is therefore 60.

4. The use of standard scale. For each large box, there is a set scale. The first box is at 300, the second at 150, the third at 100, the fourth at 75, the fifth at 60. Using the R-to-R interval, count the big boxes between two consecutive R waves. For example, there are three big boxes. Looking at the set scale, the estimated heart rate is 100.

Basically, what is being measured is the ventricular heart rate since R to R interval was used. To determine the atrial rate, use the P-to-P interval instead. If there was a P wave for every QRS complex, then there is no need to measure the P-to-P interval. It would produce the same results as with the R-to-R interval.

Checking the Atrial Contraction

Simply look at the P waves. Check if there is a P wave for every QRS complex. Check if the P waves are consistent in appearance and occurrence. Absence of P waves is an indication of an atrial contraction problem.

Checking the Ventricular Contraction

This time, assess the QRS complexes. Examine the height and the width of each complex. Measure the rhythm and rate using the R-to-R interval. Note the appearance of the complexes. Take note that QRS duration among children is shorter than adults. This is normal. However prolonged duration of QRS complexes could be indicative of hyperkalemia (excess Potassium) or bundle branch block.

As the ventricles work harder than the atria, an increase in amplitude or voltage could indicate hypertrophy (enlargement) of the ventricles. Watch out for the absence of a Q wave also, as this is an indication of a myocardial infarction – a medical condition requiring immediate attention.

Checking the Atrioventricular Conduction Time

Determine the PR interval. There should be 3 to 5 small boxes from the P wave to the next R wave. A long PR interval is indicative of a first-degree heart block or other medical conditions. A short one is oftentimes harmless and quite common especially if the person is physically active.

Checking the Ventricular Repolarization

Examine the T waves. Look at the deflections carefully. As the T wave represents ventricular repolarization, it is of utmost importance to examine this properly as the heart cannot continue without resting. These are the possible reasons for the different deflections one might see in the ECG strip.

- Flat T wave – there is hypokalemia or coronary ischemia

- Tall and narrow T wave – Indicative of hyperkalemia

- Negative T wave – could be a sign of left ventricular hypertrophy, CNS disorder or coronary ischemia.

Checking the ST Segment

Another not-to-be-missed portion to check is the ST segment. Changes in this waveform can mean many things such as:

- Depressed ST segment (with long duration and high voltage or amplitude)– ischemia

- Elevated ST segment – acute myocardial infarction

When one is very familiar with the normal values and appearance of normal ECG results, it will be easier to detect or notice any deviation from the normal. In the next chapter, learn about arrhythmias and their ECG interpretations.

Chapter 5:
Recognizing Arrhythmias

As one becomes familiar with how a normal ECG result looks, unusual tracings or irregular readings will be easy to recognize. Whether one has a medical background or not, the basic knowledge on ECG can assist them in identifying what kind of arrhythmia is on the ECG result.

Here are some common arrhythmias:

Premature Heart Beat

Premature Ventricular Contractions (PVC) - In layman's term, this is when the heart skips a beat. It is considered as the most common arrhythmia. Even healthy individuals may experience this arrhythmia once in a while. The causative factors include stress, heavy workouts, caffeine and nicotine.

On the ECG paper, the QRS complexes appear broad. The sinus impulse comes prematurely. There are deviations in the ST segment and T waves.

Tachycardia of the Atrium

1. Atrial Fibrillation. More commonly known as heart quivering, this arrhythmia, also called as Afib or AF, manifests an increased heart rate with difficulty in breathing among its sufferers. Here, the atria fails to beat effectively, leading to the pooling of blood in the upper chamber of the heart. Without proper treatment, this arrhythmia can progress to serious complications such as stroke.

On the ECG paper, there would be no P waves. The R-R intervals would be irregular. The size of QRS complexes is not uniform, too.

2. Atrial Flutter. This arrhythmia goes unnoticed for years. Why? It is because the symptoms are tolerable and appear to be normal. For example, after a heavy workout, one may feel palpitations, increased heart rate and labored breathing. These symptoms are oftentimes disregarded. Most people with cardiac diseases are afflicted with atrial flutter. However, even those with normal hearts can also acquire this. Take note though that untreated atrial flutter can lead to serious complications too such as heart failure.

   During the ECG reading, atrial rate can reach up to 300 beats per minute. The ventricular rate could be half of the atrial rate due to the body's compensation. The AV ratio is at 2:1 or 3:1. This is known as the Saw Tooth pattern. It will be impossible to measure the PR interval.

3. Supraventricular Tachycardia. This arrhythmia originates above the ventricles; hence, the prefix supra, meaning above. It could be in the atria or AV node. The person afflicted with this condition could sometimes suffer from a very fast heartbeat followed by a sudden slow heart rate.

   On the ECG strip, the atrial rate can range from 180-250 beats per minute. It is sometimes difficult to distinguish from sinus tachycardia.

Tachycardia of the ventricles

1. Ventricular Fibrillation. This arrhythmia is a medical emergency that should be attended to as soon as possible. The patient could die if VFib is not managed within minutes. Here, the ventricles make rapid, chaotic impulses leading to an inadequate supply of oxygenated blood to the vital organs.

    Usually, these types of irregular ECG readings are learned first. They are easy to recognize as both P waves and QRS complexes are not identifiable. It just looks like a wavy line. There is no rhythm, too.

2. Ventricular Tachycardia (V-tach) - This medical emergency requires immediate management. It is characterized by rapid heart rate. It results as one of the ventricles malfunctions.

    The ECG reading is easy to recognize, too. There are no P-waves. The QRS complexes are bizarre in appearance. PR intervals are immeasurable.

Bradycardia Arrhythmia

Conduction block. This arrhythmia is caused by a delay or blockage of the electrical impulses along the course of the conduction pathway. The location can be anywhere - atria, ventricles or bundle of His. In the ECG strip, there will be a regular rhythm. The P waves and PR intervals are within normal ranges and appearances. The QRS complexes are wider than normal.

Other Arrhythmias

These are just the common arrhythmias. Other arrhythmias have different tracings on the ECG paper. These may take time to learn but with patience and practice, one will be able to recognize these arrhythmias as well.

Chapter 6:
Caring for the Heart

It is one thing to be able to interpret ECG results and another thing to enjoy normal ECG readings after every checkup. This is possible when proper care of the heart is observed. Do not wait until it is too late before you start caring for the heart. By that time, it is usually too late to do anything to revive it.

As a precautionary measure, the individual should always inform the primary health care provider of the changes that he or she intends to undertake.

Here are some tips for a healthy heart.

1. Heart-healthy diet. Various studies and research have proven time and time again that fruits and vegetables are good for the heart. Unhealthy fats such as saturated and trans-fats should be avoided or totally eliminated from one's diet. Stay away from processed foods also. Here are the top 12 recommended foods that the heart will love.

    a. Yogurt

    b. Whole grains

    c. Raisins

    d. Fish/Salmon

    e. Beans

    f. Nuts

    g. Tomatoes

h. Apples

   i. Pop corn

   j. Green tea

   k. Chocolates

   l. Red wine

2. Exercise. Aside from losing the excess weight that burdens the heart, exercise also promotes good circulation of blood. Start with a basic program and progress according to the recommendations of the doctor or the trainer. Brisk walking for 15 minutes every other day is also recommended.

3. Learn to manage stress. Studies have linked stress and cardiac diseases for decades now. Inability to refrain from worrying and being anxious leads to various medical conditions for some people. There are many programs one can enroll in or take, in order to combat stress. Included are yoga, meditation, having a pet, or taking a new hobby.

4. Practicing a healthy lifestyle. Ceasing from smoking and drinking alcohol would do the heart a lot of good. Nicotine from cigarettes has been named as the culprit of most medical conditions concerning the heart. On the other hand, alcohol weakens the muscles of the heart, making it hard to pump blood all over the body. In addition, the risk of having hypertension, obesity, heart attack, and stroke is increased for those who are heavy drinkers of alcoholic beverages.

5. Adequate rest and sleep. Although the heart pumps nonstop, it needs rest, too. An individual allows the heart's cells and muscles to recuperate, recharge, reproduce, and rejuvenate when he or she sleeps for 6-8 hours a night.

6. Be merry. The old adage "laughter is the best medicine" runs true when it comes to the heart. Laughing out loud everyday can boost the health of one's heart almost the same way as exercise does.

7. Enjoying a healthy sex life. Being intimate with one's spouse is not only good for marriage, but also for the heart. One research study equates a single intercourse to a 30-minute heavy workout.

8. Living life to the fullest. One's heart will benefit a lot when there is peace, fun, and contentment in the mind and spirit. As they say, life is short to be wasted on the nonessentials of living. Make sure that each day is filled with expectations of good things to come to oneself.

To add to the list, have a regular check up. Do a routine ECG once or twice a year or as recommended by the doctor. Knowing how to do ECG interpretation is a good skill; however, having a healthy heart is much better.

Conclusion

Thank you again for downloading this book!

I hope this book was able to help you learn more about ECG interpretation!

The next step is to put the strategies provided into use, and begin interpreting ECG scans!

Finally, if you enjoyed this book, please take the time to share your thoughts and post a review on Amazon. It'd be greatly appreciated!

Thank you and good luck!

www.ingramcontent.com/pod-product-compliance
Lightning Source LLC
LaVergne TN
LVHW021746060526
838200LV00052B/3508